Craniosacral Therapy

A Beginner's Guide and Overview on Its Use Cases, with an FAQ

FELICITY PAULMAN

Disclaimer

By reading this disclaimer, you are accepting the terms of the disclaimer in full. If you disagree with this disclaimer, please do not read the guide.

All of the content within this guide is provided for informational and educational purposes only, and should not be accepted as independent medical or other professional advice. The author is not a doctor, physician, nurse, mental health provider, or registered nutritionist/dietician. Therefore, using and reading this guide does not establish any form of a physician-patient relationship.

Always consult with a physician or another qualified health provider with any issues or questions you might have regarding any sort of medical condition. Do not ever disregard any qualified professional medical advice or delay seeking that advice because of anything you have read in this guide. The information in this guide is not intended to be any sort of medical advice and should not be used in lieu of any medical advice by a licensed and qualified medical professional.

The information in this guide has been compiled from a variety of known sources. However, the author cannot attest to or guarantee the accuracy of each source and thus should not be held liable for any errors or omissions.

Introduction

Have you ever experienced a feeling that you were bearing the burden of the entire world on your shoulders? Do you experience persistent pain or stress on a regular basis? If so, you're not alone. There are a lot of people who battle with mental or physical problems that might lower their overall quality of life. Craniosacral therapy is a method that is both compassionate and successful in its approach to resolving these issues and fostering healing from the inside out.

Craniosacral therapy, in contrast to other forms of treatment such as talk therapy or touch therapy, is intended to function in conjunction with the natural healing processes of the body. This indicates that it may be useful in the treatment of a wide variety of conditions, ranging from persistent pain and stress to anxiety and depression. Additionally, it is risk-free for individuals of every age, from infants to senior citizens.

But what exactly is meant by the term "craniosacral therapy," and how does the treatment itself take place? This guide will help you out in those situations. We have compiled an extensive resource with the goal of assisting you in gaining an in-depth understanding of craniosacral treatment, including its origins, the underlying theory that underpins it, as well as its practical uses and possible advantages.

In this Guide, we will talk about the following:

- What is Craniosacral Therapy?
- Benefits of Craniosacral Therapy
- Advantages and Disadvantages of Craniosacral Therapy
- Side Effects
- How Craniosacral Therapy Works
- Common Techniques Used In CranioSacral Therapy
- Use Cases
- Step Guide To Getting Started Craniosacral Therapy Session
- What to Expect During Craniosacral Therapy
- Things To Do and To Avoid After Craniosacral Therapy

Craniosacral therapy could be just what you've been looking for if you've been looking for an approach to healing that is both non-invasive and holistic. This therapy can assist in the reduction of pain, improvement of mobility, and promotion of overall well-being by drawing on the body's innate capacity for healing.

Continue reading to find out more information about craniosacral therapy and the benefits it may have for you. This book will provide all the facts you need to make an informed decision about whether or not craniosacral therapy is suited for you, regardless of whether you are completely unfamiliar with it or have been thinking about giving it a shot for some time. Therefore, take a cup of tea, make yourself comfy, and allow me to guide you through an introduction to the field of craniosacral treatment.

Table of Contents

CHAPTER 1: WHAT IS CRANIOSACRAL THERAPY?

Craniosacral therapy is a form of bodywork that uses gentle touch to balance the craniosacral system in the body. This system includes the bones, soft tissues, and fluids that surround the brain and spinal cord.

Practitioners of this therapy believe that by releasing tension and blockages in the craniosacral system, the body can better heal itself and improve overall health and well-being. The therapy is often used to treat a variety of conditions such as headaches, neck and back pain, stress and anxiety, and sleep disturbances.

Why this beginner's guide is needed to get started with Craniosacral Therapy

This beginner's guide is needed to get started with Craniosacral Therapy because it provides an overview of what the therapy is, how it works, and what to expect during a session. Many people may be unfamiliar with this gentle technique, and may not know where to begin. This guide can serve as a starting point for those who are interested in trying Craniosacral Therapy but are unsure of what to expect.

By providing an understanding of the craniosacral system, the benefits of the therapy, and how to find a qualified practitioner, this guide can help potential clients make informed decisions about their health care. It can also help them to prepare for their first session, by giving them an idea of what will happen, what to wear, and how to communicate with the therapist.

Overall, this beginner's guide is essential for those who are new to Craniosacral Therapy and want to know more about this gentle and natural approach to healing. It can provide valuable information that can help people make informed decisions about their health, and empower them to take control of their well-being.

Background

Dr. John Upledger made the discovery of the craniosacral system after observing the spinal cord moving in a cyclical motion while aiding in an operation. This observation led to the development of craniosacral therapy. To gain a deeper understanding of the movement he had experienced, he enrolled in a class offered by The Cranial Academy. There, he came to the conclusion that the movement was connected to the cranial bones and the sacrum via the dural membranes.

Between the years 1975 and 1983, Dr. Upledger was a research fellow at Michigan State University. During that time, he led a team that established the existence of the craniosacral system and provided a model to understand the process behind it. Many disorders that affect the brain and spinal cord are not well understood, but they could be successfully treated if certain constraints in this system were corrected.

As a result of Dr. Upledger's research on the craniosacral system, new approaches to use it in the treatment of health issues that were resistant to being treated with conventional methods have been developed. His methods gradually shifted their focus to be more fluid-oriented, membrane-oriented, cellular-oriented, and energy-oriented, and they resonated with quantum physics.

In conclusion, a random occurrence that occurred when Dr. John Upledger was performing an operation led to the discovery of the craniosacral system, which he subsequently explored further while working at Michigan State University. He came up with innovative applications of the technology to treat medical conditions that did not respond to the standard treatments that were available.

Benefits of Craniosacral Therapy

There are many potential benefits of craniosacral therapy. The goal of the therapy is to improve overall health and well-being by releasing tension in the body, and it is effective at treating a variety of conditions. Here are some of the possible benefits:

- **Relieves pain**

Craniosacral Therapy targets the central nervous system to alleviate pain. By using gentle touch and specific techniques, practitioners help to release restrictions in soft tissues and improve the flow of cerebrospinal fluid, which can reduce pain and discomfort.

- **Reduces stress and anxiety**

Craniosacral Therapy is effective in reducing stress and anxiety. The therapy works by applying gentle pressure on specific points of the body, which can have a calming effect on the nervous system. This, in turn, can help reduce the levels of stress hormones in the body. Studies show that regular sessions of Craniosacral Therapy can improve overall well-being and promote relaxation.

- **Improves sleep**

Craniosacral Therapy has been known to improve sleep quality for many individuals, allowing them to have a more restful and rejuvenating sleep. This therapy achieves this by focusing on the craniosacral system, which is responsible for regulating the body's natural rhythm.

Through gentle touch, this therapy can relieve tension and help the body relax, leading to better sleep. Craniosacral Therapy can assist in reducing symptoms of insomnia, making it an effective and holistic solution for individuals struggling with sleep issues. With its non-invasive and drug-free approach, the therapy is gaining popularity as a natural alternative for improving sleep quality.

- **Boosts immune function**

Craniosacral Therapy has been found to provide immense benefits for improving the immune system's function. By reducing the levels of stress hormones and promoting relaxation throughout the body, the therapy helps to optimize the immune system's ability to fight off infections and diseases.

It is believed that by targeting the central nervous system, the therapy helps boost the production of natural killer cells, which play a crucial role in fighting off pathogenic viruses, bacteria, and other harmful microorganisms. Over time, regular Craniosacral Therapy sessions can help promote a stronger and healthier immune response, leading to better overall health and well-being.

- **Enhances overall well-being**

Craniosacral Therapy has been known to enhance one's overall well-being. Patients can experience a sense of deep relaxation, inner peace, and balance after a session. Such positive effects happen due to the therapy's impact on the central nervous system, which regulates bodily functions.

By gently manipulating the skull and spine, the therapist releases tension and facilitates the natural healing process. This kind of therapy is also beneficial for migraines, TMJ syndrome, and chronic pain. Overall, Craniosacral Therapy promotes holistic wellness by restoring the natural rhythms of the body.

- **Helps with pregnancy-related symptoms**

Craniosacral therapy is a beneficial treatment for pregnant women who experience discomfort during pregnancy. It can alleviate various pregnancy-related symptoms such as back pain, swelling, and fatigue.

This gentle manual therapy technique focuses on the craniosacral system, which encompasses the head, spine, and sacrum, and works to restore the body's natural balance. Using a light touch, the therapist can release tension and stimulate the body's natural healing process, resulting in a reduction of pain and discomfort.

- **Supports infant and children's development**

Craniosacral Therapy can be beneficial for newborn babies with birth traumas, colic, difficulty breastfeeding, or even sleeping problems. Children can also benefit from this therapy as it helps to promote healthy growth and development by addressing issues such as learning disabilities, motor coordination, behavior problems, and more.

While Craniosacral Therapy is not a substitute for medical care, it can be a complementary therapy that many individuals have found helpful for improving their overall health and well-being.

- **Side Effects**

Although Craniosacral Therapy is generally considered safe and effective, some potential side effects may occur. Some people may experience temporary discomfort or pain during the treatment as restrictions are released from the body.

Other possible side effects include;

- **Headaches**

Headaches can be a common side effect of Craniosacral Therapy. This is due to the release of tension and pressure in the head and neck, which can cause temporary discomfort for some individuals. While these headaches typically subside within a few hours, it is recommended to stay hydrated and avoid strenuous activities after a session.

However, it is important to note that not everyone experiences post-session headaches, and they do not necessarily indicate that the therapy was ineffective. Rather, they are a sign that the body is responding to the treatment and releasing pent-up stress.

- **Fatigue**

Fatigue is a common side effect of Craniosacral Therapy, a gentle technique that aims to promote relaxation and alleviate physical and emotional stress. This fatigue may be caused by the deep relaxation induced by the therapy, which can be both physically and emotionally draining. However, the fatigue is usually temporary and may indicate that the therapy is working effectively.

- **Emotional release**

Emotional release is a common side effect of Craniosacral Therapy. People may experience overwhelming emotions or memories that have been stored in their bodies. This can be positive in the long term but can be distressing for some. It is important to work with a qualified therapist who can provide emotional support and guidance throughout the process.

It is also essential to understand that emotional release is a natural and important part of the healing process, as it allows the body to release tension and trauma that may have been stored for years.

- **Nausea**

Nausea and dizziness may occur after a Craniosacral Therapy session due to the release of toxins from the body. While rare, these side effects can be a sign that the treatment is working. Clients need to drink plenty of water to help flush out these toxins and to communicate any discomfort with their therapist. In most cases, symptoms will subside within a few hours.

- **Muscle soreness**

Muscle soreness or stiffness may occur after receiving Craniosacral Therapy due to the release of tension in muscles. This effect can be temporary and is a sign that the treatment is doing its job by addressing areas of tension and imbalance in the body.

Proper hydration and gentle stretching can help ease discomfort and promote healing. It is important to communicate any discomfort to the therapist to ensure that they can adjust the treatment as needed for the client's comfort.

It's important to note that these side effects are relatively uncommon, and many people

experience no side effects at all from Craniosacral Therapy. If you have any concerns about the potential side effects of this therapy, be sure to talk to your healthcare provider. Additionally, if you experience any severe or persistent side effects after a session, seek medical attention right away.

CHAPTER 2: HOW CRANIOSACRAL THERAPY WORKS

The craniosacral system is made up of the bones, membranes, and cerebrospinal fluid that surround and protect the brain and spinal cord. This system extends from the bones of the skull, face, and mouth (the "cranium") down to the sacrum (the triangular bone at the base of the spine).

Cerebrospinal fluid (CSF) is a clear liquid that flows through the craniosacral system, providing nourishment and protection to the brain and spinal cord. This fluid fluctuates in volume and pressure, and its movement is often described as a rhythmic pulse.

Proponents of Craniosacral Therapy believe that restrictions or blockages in the craniosacral system can cause a range of physical and emotional problems. By using gentle touch and manipulation, therapists aim to release these restrictions and improve the balance and function of the craniosacral system.

Common techniques used in Craniosacral Therapy

During a Craniosacral Therapy session, the therapist will use their hands to feel for areas of tension or restriction in the craniosacral system and apply gentle pressure to help release these areas. This can help promote relaxation, reduce pain and stress, and improve overall health and well-being.

The therapist may begin the session by placing their hands on the patient's body in various positions to assess the overall state of the craniosacral system. They will then use specific techniques to release any blockages or restrictions they find.

Some common techniques used in Craniosacral Therapy include:

Still point induction

In the context of Craniosacral Therapy, Still Point Induction is a technique used to induce deep relaxation by holding a specific area of the body. This helps release tension and promotes healing. During the session, the therapist finds the still point, which is a moment of pause between the inhalation and exhalation, and holds it.

This technique creates a sense of calmness and stillness, allowing the body to restore its natural balance, which can lead to positive effects on the muscular, nervous, and immune systems. The Still Point Induction technique is a powerful tool for those seeking to reduce stress and achieve a greater sense of well-being.

Release of the diaphragms

To release tension in the diaphragms during Craniosacral Therapy, the therapist applies gentle pressure on these thin muscles that separate the chest and abdominal cavities. This technique can help to improve breathing and promote relaxation.

Relaxing the diaphragms can lead to overall tension release throughout the body, which can positively impact the musculoskeletal system. Additionally, this method can help alleviate pain and improve overall well-being. The therapist can adjust the amount of pressure applied based on the client's comfort and needs.

Fascial unwinding

In Craniosacral Therapy, fascial unwinding is a commonly utilized technique to relieve restrictions in the fascia. Through gentle movements, the therapist can promote a release of tension in the connective tissue surrounding and supporting muscles, bones, and organs.

This technique may also encourage circulation and enhance the body's natural ability to heal. Fascial unwinding is a vital component of Craniosacral Therapy, and when skillfully applied, it can help to alleviate pain and promote overall body balance and wellness.

Somatic emotional release

In Craniosacral Therapy, somatic emotional release is employed to access deep-rooted emotional patterns and memories that may be stored in the body. Through gentle touch and pressure, the therapist helps the client release stagnant emotions, promoting a greater sense of relaxation, emotional balance, and physical well-being.

This technique is based on the idea that emotional trauma can manifest in physical tension and discomfort and that by addressing these underlying emotions, the body's natural healing abilities can be activated. Somatic emotional release is particularly effective in treating conditions such as chronic pain, anxiety, and depression, and can be integrated with other therapeutic modalities to provide a comprehensive approach to wellness.

Cranial bone adjustments

In Craniosacral Therapy, cranial bone adjustments involve the use of gentle pressure to manipulate the skull and facial bones. The therapist aims to release any restrictions that may be affecting the patient's posture and alignment. The connectors between the cranial bones are quite flexible, hence any tension or misalignment can cause pressure on the brain and spinal cord leading to a range of issues.

Manipulating these bones can help to release stress on the nervous system, promoting relaxation and overall well-being. The manipulations are performed in a careful and precise manner, often with the patient remaining comfortable and relaxed throughout the process.

Visceral manipulation

In Craniosacral Therapy, the technique of visceral manipulation is applied to the organs and surrounding tissues to help release tension and promote improved organ function and overall health. This technique involves using a gentle touch to manipulate the organs and increase their mobility.

By doing so, the therapist can help reduce pain and discomfort in the body and promote healing. This therapy is particularly effective for individuals with chronic pain or inflammation, digestive issues, and other chronic conditions that impact the organs. The technique is safe and non-invasive, making it an excellent option for individuals seeking natural, alternative, and non-pharmaceutical therapies for their health concerns.

Energy work

Incorporating energy work techniques into Craniosacral Therapy sessions can enhance the balancing and healing benefits. Two examples of energy work techniques used are Reiki and chakra balancing. Reiki, a Japanese technique, involves the transfer of energy from the practitioner's hands to the client's body to promote relaxation and healing.

Chakra balancing focuses on aligning the body's seven chakras, or energy centers, to improve overall health and well-being. When combined with Craniosacral Therapy, energy work techniques may allow the client to experience a deeper sense of relaxation and balance on an energetic level.

Positional release

In Craniosacral Therapy, the positional release is used to help ease tension and pain in the body. This technique involves positioning the body in a specific way to promote relaxation and allow for the release of tension in the muscles and connective tissues. By positioning the body in a way that takes the pressure off of specific areas, a therapist can help to reduce pain and improve mobility.

This approach is often combined with other therapeutic techniques to provide a comprehensive treatment approach that addresses the underlying causes of pain and discomfort. Clients can benefit from positional release both during individual therapy sessions and through regular self-care practices designed to promote relaxation and ease tension.

By using gentle touch to release tension and blockages, Craniosacral Therapy aims to promote relaxation, reduce pain and stress, and improve overall health and well-being.

CHAPTER 3: USE CASES

Craniosacral Therapy can be useful for a wide range of physical and emotional issues. Here are some potential uses for this therapy:

Sure, here are 15 use cases of Craniosacral Therapy and their descriptions:

1. **Headaches and Migraines:** Craniosacral therapy can help treat headaches and migraines by relieving tension in the craniosacral system, which is one of the body's most important systems. This has the potential to lessen inflammation, boost circulation, and make one feel more relaxed.
2. **TMJ Dysfunction:** The mild procedures employed in Craniosacral Therapy have the potential to help patients suffering from TMJ dysfunction alleviate jaw pain and improve their function. The therapy can help restore appropriate alignment and alleviate discomfort by relieving constraints in the craniosacral system, which can be a source of tension.
3. **Back and Neck Pain:** Craniosacral therapy has been shown to be an effective treatment for back and neck discomfort. This is accomplished by releasing tension in the spine and improving the correct alignment of the

vertebrae. Because of this, one may experience less discomfort, increased mobility, and improved posture as a result.

4. **Fibromyalgia:** Craniosacral Therapy is a mild treatment that can help alleviate pain, exhaustion, and other symptoms that are linked with fibromyalgia. People who suffer from fibromyalgia may find that this therapy is beneficial to their condition.

5. **Chronic Fatigue Syndrome:** Craniosacral Therapy can be of assistance to those who suffer from Chronic Fatigue Syndrome by enhancing circulation, decreasing inflammation, and fostering calm. The therapy can help reduce fatigue and enhance overall energy levels because it addresses the underlying issues that are contributing to it.

6. **PTSD and Anxiety:** Those who suffer from post-traumatic stress disorder (PTSD) and anxiety may find that the relaxing benefits of craniosacral therapy (also known as craniosacral therapy) are beneficial. The therapy can help alleviate symptoms such as panic attacks and hypervigilance by encouraging relaxation and relieving tension in the body.

7. **Autism and ADHD:** Craniosacral therapy has been shown to be useful for children with autism and attention deficit hyperactivity disorder (ADHD) by lowering hyperactivity and enhancing focus. The soothing touch can assist calm the nervous system, which in turn helps promote more controlled conduct.

8. **Insomnia:** Craniosacral therapy is a treatment that may be helpful for people who suffer from insomnia. The therapy has the potential to improve both the quality

and quantity of sleep because it helps promote relaxation and calms the nervous system.

9. **Sinusitis:** Those who suffer from sinusitis may find relief from their symptoms by undergoing craniosacral therapy, which involves the careful manipulation of the craniosacral system. This treatment is beneficial for reducing inflammation and enhancing drainage in the sinuses.

10. **Tinnitus:** Craniosacral Therapy can be useful in lowering the symptoms of tinnitus by improving circulation and reducing inflammation. Tinnitus is caused by ringing in the ears. This can result in a reduction in the amount of sound that is experienced as well as an improvement in overall quality of life.

11. **Digestive Disorders:** Craniosacral therapy can help improve digestion by increasing relaxation and lowering tension in the digestive tract. This can help patients who suffer from digestive disorders. The symptoms of illnesses such as irritable bowel syndrome (IBS), constipation, and acid reflux may improve as a result of this.

12. **Menstrual Cramps:** Craniosacral therapy has been shown to be effective in the treatment of menstrual cramps by reducing tension in the pelvic region, which in turn improves blood flow. This therapy has the potential to provide great pain relief because it addresses the underlying causes.

13. **Post-surgical Recovery:** Because it is a non-invasive kind of treatment, Craniosacral Therapy is a great option for those recovering from surgery because it speeds up the healing process. The treatment can assist

in accelerating the healing process because it facilitates relaxation and brings inflammatory levels down.

14. **Sports Injuries:** Craniosacral therapy is an effective treatment option for athletes who are trying to recover from injuries sustained in sports. The techniques used in it are very soft, which helps to alleviate pain and inflammation and promotes a better range of motion.

15. **Stroke and Traumatic Brain Injury Recovery:** Craniosacral Therapy may be of assistance to patients suffering from a stroke or traumatic brain injury. The treatment has the potential to improve overall recovery results by enhancing circulation and decreasing inflammation.

In summary, Craniosacral Therapy can be used to address a wide range of physical and emotional conditions. From headaches and TMJ dysfunction to PTSD and stroke recovery, this gentle therapy offers many potential benefits for those seeking to optimize their health and well-being.

Advantages of Craniosacral Therapy

Craniosacral Therapy has many advantages over other forms of bodywork. Here are some of its benefits:

Non-invasive

Craniosacral therapy is a form of alternative medicine that is both mild and non-invasive. It does not include the use of any pharmaceuticals or surgical procedures. Touch and manipulation of the craniosacral system are the only components of the practice. Delicate physical techniques are used to remove constraints in the body's tissues, which are the only components of the practice. Because of this, it is a technique for healing that is both safe and natural, and there is no risk of any harmful side effects or consequences.

Personalized treatment

Each session of Craniosacral Therapy is customized to meet the specific requirements and concerns of the individual receiving it. Together with you, the therapist will analyze your craniosacral system to locate any areas of stress or restriction, and then they will devise a treatment strategy that is customized to meet the requirements of your body. This individualized strategy has the potential to assist optimize results and obtain the greatest possible advantages from treatment.

Holistic Approach

Craniosacral therapy provides a comprehensive approach to treatment, focusing not only on the patient's physical symptoms but also on the patient's mental and spiritual well-being as well. The therapy has the potential to contribute to the total well-being and equilibrium of the patient by treating the person as a whole. This can result in a higher feeling of vigor, improved mental clarity, and an enhanced capacity to deal with stress and obstacles.

Suitable for All Ages

Craniosacral therapy does not pose any health risks and has been shown to be beneficial for patients of all ages, from babies to the elderly. Athletes and senior citizens, in addition to children struggling with developmental and behavioral challenges, may find it to be of special use. Because of the therapy's non-aggressive nature, it is an excellent choice for patients who might have adverse reactions to other forms of treatment that are more aggressive.

Complementary to other therapies

It is possible to combine Craniosacral Therapy with other forms of treatment, such as Western medicine, chiropractic care, acupuncture, and massage therapy. It is possible for it to boost the effects of these therapies and provide extra benefits in terms of boosting healing and lowering pain levels. Because of this, it is a flexible and adaptable treatment that may be used in a greater variety of healthcare strategies.

In summary, each advantage of Craniosacral Therapy offers unique benefits for those seeking a gentle and natural approach to healing. Personalization, holistic care, non-invasiveness, suitability for all ages, and versatility in combination with other therapies all make Craniosacral Therapy an attractive option for those seeking to optimize their health and well-being.

Disadvantages of Craniosacral Therapy

Craniosacral Therapy is generally safe and well-tolerated, but there are a few potential drawbacks. Here are some of the disadvantages to consider:

Limited scientific research

One major disadvantage of Craniosacral Therapy is the limited scientific research supporting its effectiveness. While some studies suggest its potential benefits, such as reducing pain and improving well-being, there is still a lack of rigorous research to fully understand the therapy's limitations and efficacy.

Without such research, it is difficult for healthcare professionals to confidently recommend it to patients. Additionally, the lack of an established standard for the practice and the variability of its application further underscore the importance of continued research.

Not a substitute for medical care

Although Craniosacral Therapy can provide many benefits for the body, it is important to note that it is not a substitute for medical care. Patients who rely solely on this therapy to address their medical conditions or injuries may experience further problems if they avoid seeking professional medical help.

Craniosacral Therapy should be viewed as a complementary therapy that can support overall health and well-being, but it should never be considered a replacement for traditional medical treatment.

May not be effective for everyone

While Craniosacral Therapy can offer many benefits such as relief from stress, anxiety, and chronic pain, it may not be effective for everyone. Some people may not experience any significant improvements, while others may even experience adverse effects such as dizziness, headaches, or nausea.

It is important to note that craniosacral therapy is still considered an alternative therapy and should not be used as a substitute for medical treatment or advice from a healthcare professional.

Can be expensive

Individuals opting for Craniosacral Therapy may face the financial burden of high session costs. The therapy involves a gentle touch to address cranial and spinal imbalances, which requires the therapist to have specialized skills and training.

As a result, the cost per session can be significantly high, and multiple sessions may be needed to achieve the desired results. This disadvantage can limit access to therapy for those on a budget. However, some practitioners may offer sliding scale fees or work with insurance providers to make the therapy more accessible.

Overall, Craniosacral Therapy is a safe and non-invasive therapy that can provide many benefits for those seeking relief from pain and tension. However, it's important to remember that Craniosacral Therapy should not be used as a substitute for medical care and that more research is needed to fully understand its effectiveness.

CHAPTER 4: 5-STEP GUIDE TO GETTING STARTED CRANIOSACRAL THERAPY SESSION

If you are interested in trying Craniosacral Therapy, it's important to find a qualified therapist and prepare for your first session. In this 5-step guide, we'll walk you through everything you need to know to get started with Craniosacral Therapy, from finding a qualified therapist to preparing for your first appointment and scheduling follow-up sessions.

Step-1: Research and choose a qualified therapist

The first step in getting started with Craniosacral Therapy is to research and choose a qualified therapist. It's important to find someone who has been trained in the practice and can provide quality services.

How to Find a Qualified Craniosacral Therapist

- **Research Online:** The first step in finding a qualified Craniosacral Therapist is to research online. Look for websites and directories that list practitioners in your area. You can use search engines like Google or Bing to find relevant websites. Also, check out professional organizations such as The Upledger Institute, The Milne Institute, and The Biodynamic Craniosacral Therapy Association of North America (BCTA/NA). These organizations maintain directories of qualified practitioners who meet their standards for training and certification.

- **Referrals:** Another way to find a qualified practitioner is to ask for referrals from your friends, family members, or healthcare providers. They may be able to recommend a qualified practitioner who has experience in treating your specific condition.

- **Check Credentials:** Once you have a list of potential practitioners, check their credentials. Look for Craniosacral Therapists who have undergone formal training in the therapy. Also, check if they are certified by reputable organizations such as The Upledger Institute, The Milne Institute, or The BCTA/NA.

- **Read Reviews:** Before choosing a practitioner, read reviews from their previous clients. Check their website or Facebook page, and look for reviews on third-party websites such as Yelp or Google Reviews. Reading reviews can give you an idea of the quality of care the practitioner provides.

The Importance of Choosing a Qualified Practitioner

Choosing a qualified practitioner is critical because Craniosacral Therapy involves delicate manual techniques that require proper training and experience. A qualified practitioner will be able to properly assess your condition, develop a treatment plan that is tailored to your needs, and provide safe and effective treatment. Choosing an unqualified practitioner could potentially put your health at risk, as they may not have the necessary knowledge or experience to provide safe and effective treatment.

A qualified Craniosacral Therapist should have completed a program accredited by a reputable organization like The Upledger Institute, The Milne Institute, or The BCTA/NA. These programs typically include hundreds of hours of hands-on training in therapy, as well as coursework in anatomy, physiology, and other related subjects.

It's also important to choose a practitioner who has experience working with your specific condition. For example, if you're seeking treatment for migraines, look for a Craniosacral Therapist who has experience treating migraines.

Resources for Finding a Qualified Practitioner

The Upledger Institute: The Upledger Institute offers professional training and maintains a directory of qualified Craniosacral Therapists. You can search their directory by location or therapist name.

- **The Milne Institute:** The Milne Institute offers professional training and maintains a directory of certified Craniosacral Therapists. You can search their directory by location or therapist name.
- **The Biodynamic Craniosacral Therapy Association of North America (BCTA/NA):** The BCTA/NA is a professional organization that

maintains a directory of qualified Craniosacral Therapists who have met their standards for training and certification.

- **Referrals from Healthcare Providers:** Ask your doctor or other healthcare providers for referrals. They may be familiar with qualified practitioners in your area.

- **Online Directories:** Check out online directories such as HealthProfs, Psychology Today, or GoodTherapy. These directories allow you to search for Craniosacral Therapists in your area and filter your search based on specific criteria.

In summary, finding a qualified Craniosacral Therapist is essential for receiving safe and effective treatment. By researching, asking for referrals, checking credentials, reading reviews, and using resources such as professional organizations or online directories, you can find a qualified practitioner who can help you achieve optimal health and well-being. Remember to choose a practitioner who is properly trained and experienced, and who has a good reputation in your community.

Step-2: Schedule an appointment

To schedule an appointment for Craniosacral Therapy, the individual should contact a qualified therapist and inquire about their availability, fees, and what to expect during the session. The therapist will suggest a date and time for the person's first session. It is important to arrive on time and fully prepared to discuss any concerns or issues with the therapist.

The first session will typically involve sharing the individual's medical history and identifying any areas of the body that are experiencing discomfort or pain. The therapist will use gentle touch and pressure to manipulate the craniosacral system, release any restrictions, and promote overall health and balance. It is important to take note of any changes or improvements felt during and after the session for future reference.

Step-3: Prepare for your appointment

When getting ready for a session of Craniosacral Therapy, it is essential to put on comfortable clothing that does not restrict movement and provides unrestricted access to the parts of the body that will be worked with.

In addition, it is essential to engage in mindful relaxation and focus practices in advance of the treatment session, as these can aid deeper healing when the treatment is being administered. It is also beneficial to carry a notepad or notebook to take notes during the session and record any changes or improvements noted after the session has concluded.

Step-4: Attend your appointment

When you arrive for your session, your therapist will likely ask you some questions about your medical history, symptoms, and goals for the therapy. Then, you will lie on a massage table while the therapist uses gentle touch and manipulation techniques to stimulate your body's natural healing processes.

Step-5:Follow up and schedule additional sessions

After the first session, the therapist may recommend follow-up sessions to continue supporting the body's natural healing processes. The client needs to follow any recommendations for additional sessions and schedule them as needed to optimize the benefits of the therapy.

By following these steps, you can get started with Craniosacral Therapy and begin experiencing the benefits of this gentle and non-invasive therapy. Remember, it's important to choose a qualified therapist and be open and honest about your medical history and symptoms.

What to Expect during a Craniosacral Therapy Session

During a Craniosacral Therapy session, you can expect to work closely with your therapist to develop a treatment plan that is tailored to your individual needs and goals. In this section, we'll explore what typically happens during a Craniosacral Therapy session, from the initial consultation to the therapy itself, and what you can expect to experience along the way. By knowing what to expect, you can approach your Craniosacral Therapy sessions with confidence and ease.

Here are the things to expect during a craniosacral therapy session;

Client preparation

The client can anticipate that the therapist will employ light-touch techniques during the Craniosacral Therapy session to examine and resolve imbalances in the craniosacral system.

This system consists of the bones, tissues, and cerebrospinal fluid that surround the brain and spinal cord.

The therapist will connect with the client's body to urge it to self-correct, which will result in the client experiencing increased levels of relaxation, decreased levels of pain, and an overall improvement in their health. The use of additional support such as cushions or bolsters enables optimal comfort while remaining fully dressed ensures privacy and dignity for the patient.

Gentle touch and assessment

Craniosacral therapy involves the practitioner using light touch techniques to conduct an assessment of the craniosacral system to locate and treat any potential imbalances or blockages that may be present. They can discover regions of tension or limitation within the system and bring consciousness to those areas by analyzing the rhythm of the system.

The gentle touch helps the client achieve a profound level of relaxation and promotes the body's natural capacity to repair itself, both of which are benefits experienced by the client.

Participation from the client

Craniosacral therapy requires the client to actively participate in the process of discovering and addressing issues. This is accomplished by the client engaging in a variety of procedures, such as practicing deep breathing, concentrating on certain sensations, and moving in specific ways.

This involvement enables the therapist to obtain a deeper understanding of the client's condition and allows them to customize their treatment strategy accordingly. It also makes the client feel more comfortable discussing their issues with the therapist. When the client and the therapist collaborate, they have the potential to improve treatment outcomes and the client's well-being more generally.

Treatment that is not intrusive

Craniosacral therapy is a gentle form of bodywork that focuses on releasing tension and facilitating the body's natural ability to repair itself by manipulating the bones of the skull, spine, and pelvis. The treatment intends to improve the body's innate capacity to repair itself and to free the craniosacral system of any constraints or stress that may be present.

It can help relieve stress, alleviate chronic pain, improve sleep patterns and quality, and enhance overall well-being. The therapy is safe for people of all ages, with a gentle approach that avoids any discomfort or pain. It is a non-invasive modality that effectively addresses many conditions, from migraines and tension headaches to neck and back pain, and postoperative pain.

Emotional and physical reactions

The goal of Craniosacral Therapy is to facilitate the release of tension in the body, which can result in a variety of psychological and physiological responses. To enhance the circulation of cerebrospinal fluid, the therapist will massage the patient's skull, spine, and pelvis with a soft touch.

As a consequence of this, customers may experience feelings of warmth, tingling, or profound relaxation. The goal of the treatment is to enhance patients' general health by alleviating the pain, stress, and discomfort that are frequently brought on by tension in the body. Migraine headaches, persistent pain, and conditions associated with stress all respond favorably to this treatment.

Relaxation and rejuvenation

During the treatment, the therapist will focus on the cyclical motions of the cerebrospinal fluid, which will ultimately lead to a profound feeling of relaxation throughout the entire body. It has been discovered that the treatment can ease a broad variety of illnesses, including migraines, chronic pain, anxiety, depression, and sleep disturbances, amongst others.

In addition to these benefits, it can also help improve digestion and strengthen the immune system. This treatment does not include any risks or discomfort, and it can be administered to patients of any age.

By knowing what to expect during a Craniosacral Therapy session, you can go into your appointment feeling prepared and relaxed. It's important to remember that everyone's experience with this therapy may be different, so be sure to communicate with your therapist throughout the session and let them know if you have any questions or concerns.

Things to Do After The Craniosacral Therapy

The effects of Craniosacral Therapy are cumulative, meaning that with each session you will experience greater relief from your symptoms. To maximize the benefits of your therapy sessions, it's important to take care of yourself and make lifestyle changes to support your body's natural healing processes. Here are some things you can do after Craniosacral Therapy;

- **Drink plenty of water:** It's important to drink plenty of water after a Craniosacral Therapy session to help flush out any toxins that may have been released during the session.

- **Rest and relax:** Take time to rest and relax after your session. Avoid strenuous activity or exercise for at least 24 hours.

- **Pay attention to your body:** Take note of any changes or sensations you may be feeling after your session. This can give you a better understanding of how your body is responding to the therapy.

- **Follow any recommendations from your therapist:** Your therapist may recommend specific exercises or stretches to help support your body's natural healing processes. It's important to follow these recommendations to get the most out of your therapy.

- **Schedule follow-up sessions:** Depending on your needs, your therapist may recommend follow-up sessions to help support your body's natural healing processes. Be sure to schedule these sessions as needed.

By following these steps, you can help support your body's natural healing processes and get the most out of your Craniosacral Therapy session. It's important to remember that while Craniosacral Therapy can be a helpful addition to a treatment plan, it should not be used as a substitute for medical care. If you have any questions or concerns about your therapy, be sure to talk to your healthcare provider.

Things to Avoid after Craniosacral Therapy

Just like certain things can help maximize the benefits of Craniosacral Therapy, there are also some activities and habits you should avoid after a session. Here are some things to avoid after a Craniosacral Therapy session;

- **Strenuous activity:** After a Craniosacral Therapy session, it's important to avoid strenuous physical activity for at least 24 hours. This allows your body time to rest and recover after the therapy.

- **Caffeine and other stimulants**: Avoid caffeine and other stimulants, such as energy drinks or sugary foods, after your session. These can interfere with your body's natural healing processes and may make it difficult to relax.

- **Alcohol and drugs:** It's important to avoid alcohol and drugs, including prescription medications that may cause drowsiness or impair cognitive function, after your session. These can interfere with your body's natural healing processes and may negate the benefits of the therapy.

- **Overstimulation:** After a Craniosacral Therapy session, it's important to avoid overstimulation from loud noises, bright lights, or other sensory experiences. This can help promote a sense of relaxation and calm, allowing your body to fully benefit from the therapy.

- **Stressful situations:** It's important to avoid stressful situations after your session, as this can interfere with your body's ability to relax and heal. Instead, take time to rest and practice self-care, such as taking a warm bath or engaging in meditation or deep breathing exercises.

By avoiding these things after your Craniosacral Therapy session, you can help support your body's natural healing processes and get the most out of your therapy. If you have any questions or concerns about what to avoid after your session, be sure to talk to your healthcare provider.

Conclusion

Congratulations! Congratulations, you've made it to the final section of our in-depth tutorial on Craniosacral Therapy! You are now aware of what this kind of therapy is, how it works, what to expect during a session, how to find a trained therapist, and a great deal more information.

Craniosacral Therapy can be used to treat a broad variety of ailments, ranging from physical pain to mental anguish. Hopefully, this guide has provided you with a better understanding of the benefits of Craniosacral Therapy and how it can be used to do so. You will be able to take charge of your health and wellness and find new methods to boost your general quality of life if you consult with a competent Craniosacral Therapist.

Craniosacral Therapy is a very customized form of treatment, which is one of the most important things to keep in mind regarding this type of therapy. Because it is geared toward assisting your body in its own natural healing processes, each session will be individualized to meet your specific requirements and objectives. When it comes to Craniosacral Therapy, this indicates that there is no "one size fits all" answer; rather, your therapist will work closely with you to build a treatment plan that is customized to meet your specific needs.

Craniosacral therapy might not be the best option for everyone, but it's definitely something you should look into if you're struggling with conditions like persistent pain, stress, or anything else that's lowering the quality of your life. Your entire health and well-being, as well as your ability to start experiencing life to the fullest, can be improved if you start by providing your body with the support and care it requires.

If you are considering giving Craniosacral Therapy a shot, it is imperative that you conduct adequate research in order to locate a certified therapist who possesses the required qualifications, training, and expertise. It is important to keep an open line of communication with your therapist throughout the duration of your sessions and to practice patience during the healing process. The power of Craniosacral Therapy can help you reach a greater sense of balance and well-being, but it takes time and attention on your part to make this happen.

I am appreciative of your attention to detail in reading this manual. We hope that you have found it to be enlightening, interesting, and empowering. Keep in mind that the state of your health and well-being is entirely under your control, and there are a variety of resources at your disposal to assist you in accomplishing your objectives. So get out there and show everyone that you're the boss; you've got this!

FAQ

1. What is craniosacral therapy?

Craniosacral therapy is a style of bodywork that is mild, non-invasive and focuses on balancing the craniosacral system. This system consists of the bones, fluids, and membranes that surround the brain and spinal cord. Craniosacral therapy was developed in the 1970s. Techniques using a light touch are used to alleviate tension and constraints that have built up in the body.

2. How does it work?

The therapist is able to evaluate the rhythm of the craniosacral system and discover any imbalances or blockages by making use of procedures that only require a gentle touch. They then employ gentle techniques in order to alleviate tension and encourage the body's innate capacity for healing.

3. What are some of the advantages of undergoing craniosacral therapy?

Craniosacral treatment can assist in the alleviation of physical discomfort, the reduction of stress and anxiety, the promotion of relaxation, the improvement of sleep, and the fortification of the immune system. Migraines, back discomfort, and TMJ issues are just some of the ailments that can benefit from its use.

4. What exactly takes place during a session of craniosacral therapy?

The client remains completely clothed while lying on a massage table during the session, during which the therapist uses techniques using gentle touch to locate and correct imbalances in the body. As the client's body releases tension and toxins, the client may experience sensations in either their body or their emotions.

5. Is the cranial-sacral therapy that I receive safe?

Craniosacral treatment is completely risk-free and does not involve any intrusive procedures. It is the client's choice whether or not to continue with the treatment, and they are free to discontinue it or make adjustments at any moment.

6. Who is a good candidate for receiving craniosacral therapy?

Craniosacral treatment is beneficial for a wide range of people, including individuals who suffer from chronic pain, tension, anxiety, or trouble sleeping. Additionally, persons recuperating from traumas or surgical procedures can benefit from it.

7. How many appointments do we need to schedule?

The number of sessions required varies from person to person depending on the individual's particular concerns and requirements. Although some people may feel better after just one session, for others it may take multiple sessions before they notice a meaningful change in their condition. Your therapist can assist in determining the treatment strategy that will work best for you.

References and Helpful Links

Mann, J. J., & Coeytaux, R. R. (2007). Migraine and Tension-Type Headache. In Elsevier eBooks (pp. 143–156). https://doi.org/10.1016/b978-1-4160-2954-0.50018-1

History of Craniosacral Therapy. (n.d.-b). https://iacst.ie/history-craniosacral-therapy

Professional, C. C. M. (n.d.). Craniosacral Therapy. Cleveland Clinic. https://my.clevelandclinic.org/health/treatments/17677-craniosacral-therapy

Ughreja, R. A., Venkatesan, P., Gopalakrishna, D. B., & Singh, Y. P. (2023). Feasibility and Efficacy of Craniosacral Therapy on Sleep Quality in Fibromyalgia Syndrome: a Pre-Post Pilot Trial. International Journal of Therapeutic Massage & Bodywork: Research, Education, & Practice, 16(2), 4–11. https://doi.org/10.3822/ijtmb.v16i2.819

Ehlers, A., & Clark, D. (2008). Post-traumatic stress disorder: The development of effective psychological treatments. Nordic Journal of Psychiatry, 62(sup47), 11–18. https://doi.org/10.1080/08039480802315608

Smith, L. (2023, June 7). Lymphatic Drainage Therapy with Chiropractic Care & Craniosacral Therapy in New York City. Craniosacral Therapy NY. https://www.craniosacraltherapyny.com/constipation-relief-with-chiropractic-care-craniosacral-therapy/

Castro-Sánchez, A. M., Lara-Palomo, I. C., Matarán-Peñarrocha, G. A., Saavedra-Hernández, M., Pérez-Mármol, J. M., & Aguilar-Ferrándiz, M. E. (2016). Benefits of Craniosacral Therapy in Patients with Chronic Low Back Pain: A Randomized Controlled Trial. Journal of Alternative and Complementary Medicine, 22(8), 650–657. https://doi.org/10.1089/acm.2016.0068

Massage, M. (2020). Craniosacral Therapy Massage: Fighting Insomnia with a Gentle Touch. Myotherapy Healing Massage Clinic. https://www.myohealingmassage.com/fighting-insomnia-craniosacral-therapy-massage/#:~:text=But%20you%20can%20break%20the,regulating%20our%20sleep%2Dwake%20transitions.